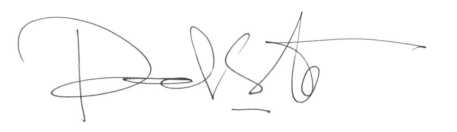

The David Starr Beauty Book

Unequalled Eyebrows

Published by BBz, LLC

Hardbound First Edition 2003

Library of Congress Control Number: 2003104114

ISBN 0-9740406-0-6

Production Manager: Edward Russell

Editors: Janet Newcomb & Eric Akin
Editorial Assistant: **Michael Wolfington**
Graphic Design & Layout: **Loren Wilson**
Illustrations: **David Starr**
Photo David Starr: **Ethan Kaminski**

Table of Contents

Foreword

Much of what David Starr writes about speaks volumes about who he is. He is confident, masterful, wickedly humorous, complimentary, observant, nurturing, intuitive, psychologically savvy, spiritual, and most of all, he is a straight shooter. He zeros in and cuts through like a laser beam to the heart of the matter. Personally, this is what I love about David Starr. He is not only authentic; he is genuinely superb in the truthful delivery of his messages. As a woman, you know it because you can feel it and sense it.

Mr. Starr understands women from the inside out. He is so psychologically in tune that I believe it is what makes his approach so unique. He is truly gifted in his vision of what it takes to bring out the best in a woman. While he knows his work about making women more beautiful, he also elicits the true essence of the heart of a woman, when she is open to it. He can be the channel to facilitate the love of self.

Many women are shy and uncomfortable around people, other women, and particularly men.

Mr. Starr is a man that many women can trust and begin a genuine dialogue about their deepest, innermost thoughts and wishes about being lovelier, not just physically, but emotionally and psychologically as well.

As a trained professional in clinical psychology, I could be arrogant and think that I know it all. However I do prefer to keep an open mind and listen to other experts.

Lucky for me, one day, Mr. Starr made some casual suggestions to me (unsolicited, of course) about how I could update my look. A light bulb went off in my head. What he pointed out were things that never occurred to me. Oh sure, I thought of these things as they related to other women, not me. I had no clue that my then current look was outdated back to the seventies. I thought to myself, no friend of mine ever pointed this out to me. They were probably afraid to incur my wrath.

That is when I realized that Mr. Starr was also very courageous because it is a very delicate matter to bring to a woman's attention that her look could be improved. This process could shatter one's ego, but the way Mr. Starr delivered his message was with respect and subtlety. Thank goodness I was not one to be hit over the head with a sledge hammer. The action that I took after a session with him literally transformed me. It was not only the changes I made in my physical appearance, but more so in my attitude about myself. I began to take better care of me; my mood, my appearance, my health.

I'm still a work in progress but I have to say that I feel more sensual, more feminine, softer, more self-assured than at any time in my teens and twenties when I had what I know now as a knock-out body and exotic looks. I couldn't even appreciate it because at that time, I tried to be invisible. I had little to no confidence.

When I was in my twenties, a man on the street stopped me and told me I was built like a brick sh*t house, I thought he was insulting me. I was not able to take compliments, no matter how raw they were.

Through out the years, I learned what it meant to be gracious. Being gracious teaches you to learn to be less judgmental and more accepting of others as well as yourself. This gives you tremendous relief and peace of mind. You don't have to continuously strive for perfection, but excellence instead, that is more consistently achievable.

In our youth pursuing society, we fight aging with a vengeance. What I love about what David Starr teaches is that you take what you have and make the most of it and the rest is a matter of attitude. I consciously and actively choose to move through the rest of my life with grace. I would not trade places with the me of twenty or thirty years ago. I like who I am and value what I know of me today because I earned my beauty and wisdom with every experience and challenge that I faced. I have the wrinkles and bulges to prove it.

Edward Russell, the financial wizard and David Starr's partner in BeautyBoyz plays a significant role in the transformation of women as well. He is so nurturing and safe to be with as you are transforming.

Remember, he is the one you come in contact with when you are vulnerable and more in touch with the newest layer of the real you. He connects with you.

He is genius in his approach to sales of BeautyBoyz products. He doesn't sell you! Can you imagine that? He just gently asks you if you need any additional items aside from what was recommended. He takes the thinking out of it for you by asking the right questions for your needs. He offers no pressure, no gimmicks, no sales pitch, no hustle. You feel respected and cherished.

You feel so good when you're leaving the studio that you just want to make sure you're not leaving anything behind, except the outdated you. It is truly a BeautyBoyz experience that can be a turning point in your life whether you're 20 or 60 years young. I highly recommend it.

Sheila Newton, Ph.D.

Clinical Psychologist

Beverly Hills, CA

On Magic and Miracles

I believe in magic and miracles. I say this because my life has been genuinely blessed with both.

I would love for you to believe in magic too. I would love for you to awaken each day expecting a miracle. And you know, all you have to do is be willing.

We all learned about magic and miracles in fairytales when we were children. If we recall the stories of Snow White and Cinderella we are instantly returned to enchantment, where miracles happen, magic occurs and dreams come true. We live happily ever after.

The story of Cinderella is filled with magic, that's why we love it. Cinderella was naturally beautiful because she was authentic. Her loving spirit beckoned her Fairy Godmother to appear. Cinderella's total self-acceptance created the magic to transform rags into a ball gown. Her state of grace changed Cinderella into the most beautiful woman in the land. She got the Prince.

The decision to be beautiful attracts the beautiful. It's all a state of perception and self-permission. Yet I hear so many women say, "When I lose thirty-pounds I will buy some nice clothes and start getting out." "When I land an important job, I'll take the time." "When Mr. Right comes along I'll slap on some lipstick, I have potential."

Well, life is filled with potential. But being beautiful takes more than potential; it takes commitment, energy and a hint of magic. One must learn to have a consciousness of beauty. You don't have to be a certain weight, or have a specific job or be with the ideal partner to show up 100 per cent. To show up, all you have to do is drop the belief that you must appear to be someone you aren't.

Showing up real gives you authenticity and energy. Energy brings out your inner beauty. Put out some energy and you are a magnet! But like Snow White, some of you have swallowed the poison apple of self-doubt, abandoned your energy and gone to sleep.

But I know how to awaken you from this sleep. My magic is simple: I see only beauty. I tell a woman how beautiful she is. I create a space for her to hear what I say. And I let her know I only say what I believe. Only what I see with my own two eyes.

Sometimes when I compliment a woman, she will correct me with, "I have so many lines!" "My makeup is a mess." "I'm so fat!" Just accept the compliment. Learn to be gracious. Being able to say "Thank you" honors the person giving the compliment and allows them to continue on their pathway.

When a woman is willing to believe in herself she moves to a very special place where miracles occur. And a miracle is, quite simply, a shift in perception. And that shift to a belief in your own beauty leads to self-acceptance and ultimately fills the void of diminished self-esteem, distorted self-image and feelings of invisibility. And the only way to be beautiful is to be willing to be beautiful.

I have always been able to perceive what women really need, not just what they think they need or want. It is a visceral, ESP sort of thing for me.

When I look into clients eyes I feel magic and see her inner self. This allows me to interpret exactly what will look best. Then I call on my experience to explore the face and do what needs to be done *correctly*. No guesswork.

As a makeup session progresses, I see a snoozy Snow White turn into a scintillating Cinderella. When I unveil the beauty that has been hiding, it's like a butterfly bursting forth from a cocoon. When a woman realizes she is genuinely beautiful, a lasting transformation occurs.

It takes tremendous strength to step forward and remove the obstacles that prevent the emergence of the real you: your resume, past choices, what you think you know, pride, family history, embarrassment, fears. But when it's done, it's well-worth the struggle and the result is incredible beauty.

Some women will simply assert, "I don't have time." If Cinderella had said to her Fairy Godmother "I don't have time for the ball." the story would have been a whole lot different. So I don't acknowledge the "I don't have time excuse."

You would never say, "I don't have time to shower," or "I don't have time to put gas in the car," or "I don't have time to pick up my ten-million dollars at Lotto." It's like anything important, you make time. The result of making time is a more visible and beautiful you; where you enter the magic kingdom of self-confidence. And real self-confidence is not arrogance, it is acceptance.

So let's take a step toward this magic kingdom of beauty. The path is right there on your face. This pathway is the key to expression. Once I tell you what it is you will be surprised and say, "Oh, I knew that." It's right there in plain view, your eyebrows. The most important part of your face and when refined and made up correctly, you need do little else.

This may seem unlikely to some of you, but it's true. In some circles, beautiful eyebrows are referred to as the "gull in flight." Beautiful, free, graceful and enchanting to view.

Eyebrows make your face. I cannot be more insistent on this point.

A Beautiful Brow

A beautiful brow describes the face in a responsive and gracious way. Eyebrows tell everyone what emotions you are currently experiencing. If you are jubilant, the brows rise for the occasion. Just as if you are angry, the brows furrow and impart that attitude as well.

Since we all want to be loved it is best to look as though we are receptive to it. When you are open to love you are your most visible. I believe eyebrows to be a cornerstone in the avenue of communication. So why not communicate a positive message. Some eyebrow shapes I have seen are not only not alluring, but they also discourage personal contact.

The importance of eyebrows became even more apparent recently. I was giving a lecture to a group of professional makeup artists. The model of the evening was a zaftig strawberry-blonde in her early fifties. The artist who brought her was eager to make her over: "I want to hide her tired skin, cover up her age spots, hide her pink undertones, and bring out her eyes."

The woman wore little makeup. The only possible weakness I saw was how she had neglected her eyebrows.

"What if I could improve your appearance by introducing you to one new thing?" I questioned. "I would be grateful," said she. So I restructured her eyebrows. While the process took place, the room was filled with "oohhs and aahhs." When finished the woman was ebullient, "I look like I have had a face lift!" "I can't believe it." It was true. She looked totally redone.

The students in the class were dumbfounded. They saw it with their own eyes, but found it hard to comprehend. Just changing the eyebrows and doing some eyebrow makeup did more than all the cover-ups in the world. When the eyebrows work, it all works.

When a woman begins to see the importance of perfectly shaped eyebrows she is astounded. The joyous proclamations include, "Why didn't anyone show me this before?" "I can't believe how incredible I look!" "I have had my brows waxed by experts but you did magic!"

Jodi wrote from Germany, "Thank you for giving me my eyebrows back....what a difference it makes!" These accolades make my work worthwhile.

Vogue wrote in 1989: "Believe it or not at his San Francisco Makeup Salon, David Starr's specialty is eyebrows." That was well before anyone considered eyebrows important to the face. Eyebrows have always been my focal point. I know perfectly shaped eyebrows are paramount to a beautiful face. My eyebrow architecture is a function of anatomy. I invented the term *eyebrow architecture©* in 1982 to explain a very special process. It is something I have studied my entire life--first with my painting and portraiture, then with cosmetology and finally with a complete study of cosmetic surgery.

It brings me great gratification to see a woman who was tentative begin to reveal her delight. That light beams brighter and brighter as each woman sees the remarkable difference. The diversity between a perfect eyebrow and a poor one is astonishing. But you have to be willing to try.

I have spent an inordinate amount of time culling and editing this panoply of information. Once you understand what to look for, you will see the difference for yourself. You can be confident because you are perfect. Confidence translates to beauty.

Confidence keeps you from being invisible. Confidence attracts others. Confidence makes you comfortable to be with.

When you are confident you appear to be in a very special place; a place where everyone will want to join you.

All you have to do is be willing to look at yourself. Be willing to rediscover yourself. Be willing to reinvent yourself. Believe that someone else can make you more beautiful than you can. While you have made up your face, I have made up thousands.

If you keep doing the same things you will always get the same results. Aren't you tired? Just let the magic happen. Everyone will want to be near the most beautiful woman in the room and it will be you!

Six Thoughts on Eyebrows:

- The entire face drops as we age; brows tilt and lower. A brow that once grew up will now grow out. The brow hairs change texture and color.

- Squeezing the muscle between the eyes alters the face and ultimately wrinkles your brow shape. If the brow is over-tweezed it causes the head of the brow to look like the top of a comma around the eye. If you have any lines or puffs they are made dramatically more obvious.

- Very often when brow hairs are tweezed or shaved they do not grow back. The legendary Lana Turner complained that the studio shaved her eyebrows and they never grew back.

- Brow colorization is best done with layers of different colors and products. Better than plain pencil or a tattoo.

- Eyebrow shape can take 10 years off your age or add 20.

- Anyone can wax an eyebrow.

The Dorsal Radix Dome*

This principle is quite important to the brow shape and described best as an imaginary line that traces the eyebrow from the lateral end of the brow to the nasal end; then down the side of the nose bone without changing its soft continuous contour. It means that the eyebrow line always guides the viewer's eye down the side of the nose, not into the orbit or eye socket.

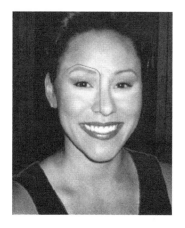 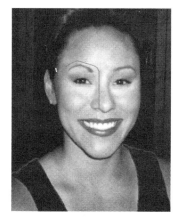

Perfect

This brow supports the entire structure of the face.

Flawed

This brow points into the eye socket and distorts the face.

*Powell & Humphreys, Proportions of the Aesthetic Face, Thieme-Stratton, Inc. 1984

The Aesthetic Triangle & Mid-Face Contour

This principle suggests there is an inverted triangle in the center of the face.   It extends from the chin to the lateral side of each eye, with an invisible line on top to form the triangle. The area inside the margins is called the Mid-Face Contour. This is what people see initially when they look at you. The eyebrows should not impede the open look of the mid-face contour.

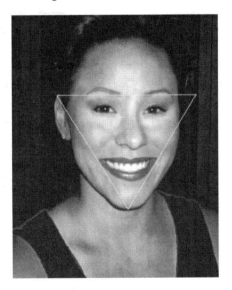

The Aesthetic Triangle

The David Starr
Eyebrow Architecture Graph©

Consider now that an eyebrow looks first-rate if it has a relationship to the structure of the face. This graph will help you envision a beautiful new eyebrow. The David Starr Eyebrow Architecture Graph© will also help you to do your brows symmetrically. "Eyeballing it," doesn't work.

By graphing you have no guess work. You can take your time and appreciate what you are creating. The result is far superior to "here a tweeze, there a tweeze," while looking down into a magnifying mirror.

When you graph your eyebrows, look straight into a mirror (standing about two feet away) so you can see the big picture. The result is far better. You will see yourself the way others see you.

You may wish to take a moment to review *Terminology* in the back of the book. (p.49)

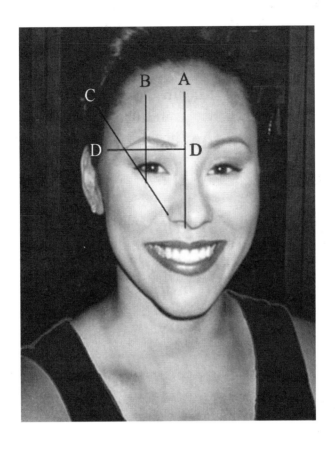

David Starr Eyebrow Graph©

The brow must begin at A.
Arch softly at B.
Terminate at C.
It must also begin and end on the same plane D.

To look great the brow must begin at A, arch softly at B, terminate at C. It must also begin and end on the same plane D.

The brow must move gracefully from thicker to thinner with no sudden or sweeping swan movements. The brow has a better feeling to it if the nasal edge of the head and lateral edge of the tail are a bit gauzy. The brows look best if you pay close attention to movement. The only arch will be the soft one at point B, nowhere else.

Study the graph on the previous page. Being familiar with a perfect eyebrow shape puts it in your consciousness.

I do suggest you use a white pencil or guide, marked on your face to achieve symmetry. Please don't do it in the car. Relax, take your time. You're worth it.

Eyebrow Positioning

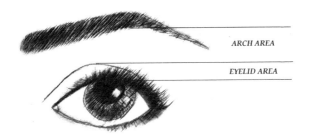

From the base of the lash to the crease of the lid should be one half the distances that exists between the crease and the highest point of the arch. The other way to envision it is that the distance between the highest point of the arch and the crease of the eyelid is twice the distance that exists between the crease and the lash base. This gives you a general guide to eyebrow positioning. Is yours too high, too low or would it look better thicker or thinner?

Example: If the lid were ½ inch wide, then from the crease to the arch would be 1 inch wide.

Look straight into a mirror with your chin parallel to the floor.

The Eyebrow Plane

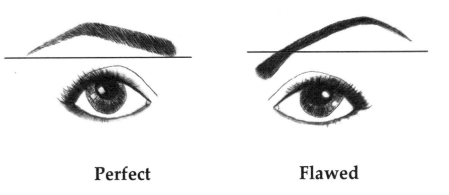

Perfect   **Flawed**

It is suggested that the eyebrow begin and end on the same plane. This means that the head of the brow and the tail must be at the same level when you are looking straight in a mirror with your chin parallel to the floor.

Brows that have been arched so the head of the brow is much lower than the rest of the structure may have moments of drama but, overall, it looks harsh.

The Eyebrow Size

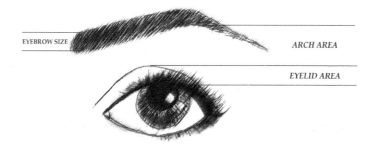

Once you have determined eyebrow position, consider the width of the brow. Generally the brow head is the thickest part of the aesthetic brow and it should be 1/3 the width of the arch area. So if the arch area is one inch, the brow would be 1/3 inch at the thickest part. If the eyelid is small, shadowing the crease (or fold) may decrease the look of the arch area.

Anatomy of an Eyebrow
The Eyebrow Contour and Profile

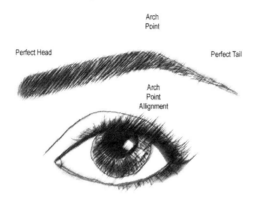

The eyebrow looks most pleasing when it makes a soft movement from thicker to thinner. No bows, no swoops and no extreme egg shapes at the arch. No pencil line tails. No sharp arch point. Fashion may suggest thicker or thinner, but the silhouette, profile or contour is always defined as what looks best on your own face.

The Eyebrow Arch

The arch of the eyebrow is proportionate to the structure of the face. When it arches gently over an imaginary vertical line measured at the lateral ring of the iris, it looks best. A soft glide that gently echoes the shape of the eye opening presents best. No sharp points. An arch can be any change or indentation in an otherwise smooth movement. What I see most often is a blurry block-like head, then an exaggerated arch with a swooping swan finish.

The Eyebrow Head

The head of the eyebrow is a fluid shape that does not have a theatrical change in contour or thickness as it travels to the arch. To curve the straight profile of the head, guides the viewer's eye into the eye socket. That makes you look like you have rings around your eyes. A bulbous or drooping head may not be as dreadful on an immaculate young face, but it certainly is for the face with grown-up age lines. The vertical nasal-edge can be straight, less dense or slightly slanted toward the nose and still be attractive.

The Eyebrow Tail

The tail of the eyebrow begins at the arch and ends with a soothing point. That point is generally directed to the top of the external auditory canal. It must not look as though if the tail continued it would drop down to your jaw. Alternately, it should not look as though if it continued it could fly off your head like an antenna. (As a side note: the tail of the brow also looks best when it echoes the top line of the upper lip.) The end of the tail should finish gently as though airbrushed to a point.

When shaping, most women make the mistake of leaving the tail with a tiny wedge of hair on it. If the arch and descent is too steep it will not be long enough to end on the same plane with the head. Conversely, if the drop is too flat it will have the problem of looking too much like a landing strip.

The First Challenge

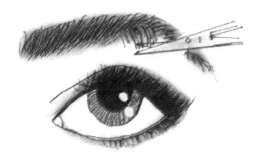

Many women tweeze their brows when they look unkempt. The problem is really length, not width. Simply put, the brow hairs are too long.

My solution is eyebrow trimming. A beautiful brow line can be achieved by simply "cutting" brow hairs that are too long. Tweezing underneath the brow growth makes the brow look wiry, unruly and at the same time too thin.

Often when hair is tweezed, it doesn't grow back. Remember the face you have today will change.

As your facial skin loses elasticity or moves with facial expression, so do your eyebrows. Exaggerated tweezing can be woefully painful as you age. I see it all the time.

It is easier to trim or base trim. As a general rule, the brow hair length must not be longer than the width of the brow base. This is very important to micro-thin brows.

Using an eyebrow groomer, comb the hairs up and gently trim off any hairs that extend higher than the base from which they grow. Comb them down and repeat the process. The brow hairs should now lie flat and look groomed. You may repeat this process as necessary. Use micro or medical scissors. Be very, very careful.

I also use BBz Micro Scissors to trim off any fine facial hair. I lay the shears flat against the skin. This makes the brow line clean and neat.

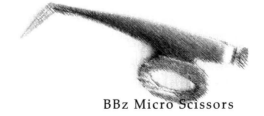

BBz Micro Scissors

The Biggest Challenge of All

Let me start with what I see as the biggest challenge to conquer. There is a fashion trend of nearly every woman I see. That is to whittle the eyebrows into a circular pattern. To shape the brow head like a cumbersome comma pointing down into the eye area. This turns the eye socket into a crater in the face and the result is unflattering. You can fix this.

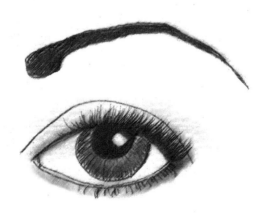

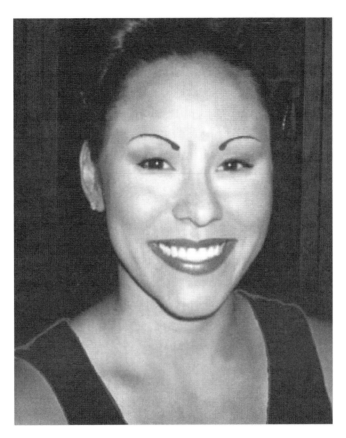

Challenged Brows

Because of Megan's natural beauty, it's easy to overlook how unappealing her eyebrows are here.

The Challenged Brow

Correcting the Brow Shape

The heavy head drop is the most common problem I see. Our goal is to make a challenged brow look more aesthetic. Your individual brow may not be as misshapen as this one. But these guides will work just the same.

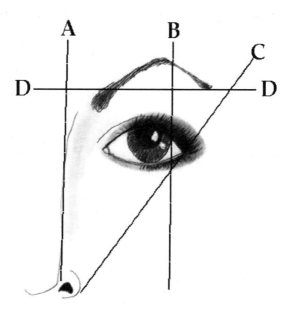

Connecting the Top Dots

A New Brow is Born

Using a brow pencil, place a dot about 1/8 inches *above* the A & D junction. Next place a dot about 1/16 inches *above* your eyebrow at the B junction. Make a third dot about 1/16 inch *above* the C & D junction. Connect the dots with straight lines.

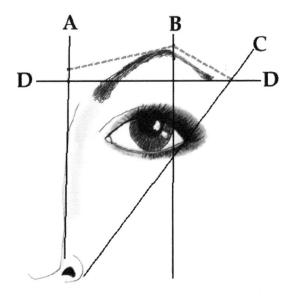

Shaping the Bottom Contour

Make a dot *on* the A & D junction. Make a second dot at B about 1/8 inch *below* the first B dot. Now make a dot at the junction of C & D. Connect the dots with straight lines. In this example we have removed the hair that fell outside of the graph.

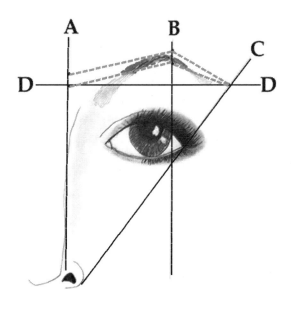

A Beautiful New Brow Contour

Now, all you have to do is fill in with color. You can use this graph if your brow is droopy, too arched, too straight or too thick. The results are always unequalled. You can thicken or thin as you prefer.

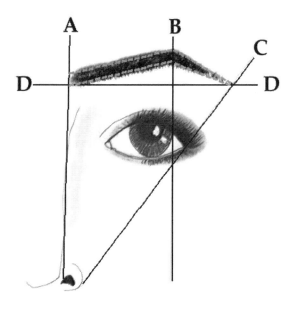

How to Makeup Your Eyebrows

Eyebrow makeup isn't just a pencil anymore. The fashionista, business tycoon, socialite or homemaker needs at least a basic understanding of how to do eyebrow makeup. Here is where you will learn how to color, highlight and makeup your eyebrows to enrich them and impact your overall appearance for the better.

Most women have spent very little time on eyebrow makeup techniques, learning something new will be an adventure. The result will be a more beautiful you. Magnificent brows make the need for other makeup far less crucial. Trust me on this one. Women come from all over to have me analyze, correct and teach them to colorize and makeup their eyebrows.

If you are one of the ladies whose brows have been tattooed on in a shape that you now find to be unappealing, they can be lasered off by a skilled professional. Some will fade with age.

Before You Color

When using a pencil to color your brows

Getting the color onto the brow is just as important as where you apply it. If you are using a pencil I prefer long very light strides. No flipper movements. No touch and go. I place the light colored pencil at the A point then tenderly and evenly proceed to B then to C. I gradually build up the color. The result is unequalled.

If you use a rub, whip or feathered motion your brow looks messy and amateurish. Also consider, this is *your* painting; proceed with poise and confidence. Polish the look for a beautiful patina. Remember, not all areas of the brow have to be the same level of darkness or lightness. Sometimes the outer most areas look better when they are lighter than the center of the brows. Gauzy.

When using a brush to color your brows

I place the tip of my brush firmly into a brow color powder. The brush will pick up the color for a beautiful transfer. But before I take the brush to the brow, I wipe out any excess on a white paper towel.

This implodes the color into the brush. The outside edges are clean, but the inside is rich with pigment. You are ready to create perfection.

In my studio I use our exclusive Brow Shaper Trios that have two different brow color powders and a wax center.

Sometimes I will first apply wax to the brow; the same soft movement from A to B to C. Then I apply the powder separately. Sometimes I will mix wax & powder for dimension. But I always wipe out the excess powder from the brush onto a paper towel.

To remove excess color from the brush; run the brush against the paper towel and make several four to six inch strokes on the paper towel. This is repeated until the paper starts to look clean. However when you bring this brush to the brow, the color that is still inside the brush will transfer where you apply it. The marvelous thing is it will look velvety, natural and slightly transparent.

When the brow looks penciled on, it looks sharp and unyielding. The result is far less attractive than the one described above.

Beautiful Natural Brows
Four easy steps to coloring brows

The coloring process is done after you know what
needs to be repaired. Visualize what you want. Then
visualize again. With this vision in mind you can
superimpose the right brow shape over a weak brow
shape. Then correct it with layers of color.

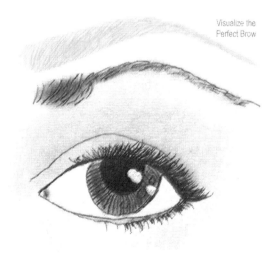

Visualize the
Perfect Brow

Step 1: Paint in the first brow powder over pencil or wax

Begin with a pencil or wax to apply a base to the skin. I have a brow shape in my vision. I move A to B, then B to C. I do not try to get a lot of color transfer with each pass. I gradually build up color. Color on color makes dimensional color. I begin with a lighter color pencil than most women expect; a blonde or taupe; for dark complexions medium brown.

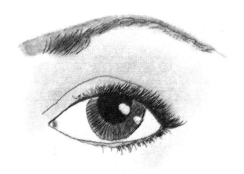

This fills in the top contour of the brow. I usually over coat the pencil or wax with a light shade of powder. In my studio I have Brow Shaper Trios. But you can use a light matte brow or shadow color.

Step 2: Paint in the second brow powder shape

This step brushes the bottom contour into place. I apply a deeper color paying very close attention to the A to B, B to C movement. My goal is to get dimension. A change in color tone can be achieved by mixing a warm and cool color.

I use a small sable slant tip brush to apply the powder. When I apply the deeper tone, I pay attention to the bottom contour line and the nasal edge of the head. This gives the brow a gauzy look.

If the brow is not strong enough, I reapply the top and bottom contour, mixing the two colors until they look natural.

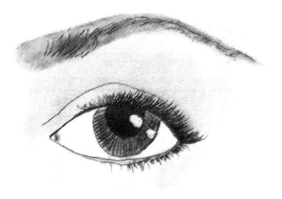

Step Three: Highlight the brow bone

I now highlight the brow bone with Alabaster Primer. It has a matte finish. I apply it with a synthetic brush in one continuous stroke with a firm motion. The brow bone is highlighted and the lower contour of the desired brow shape is more visible. For evening I trace gently over the Alabaster with a luminous shine shadow in Willow White, Pink Cream, Pale Taupe or Asteroid Silver.

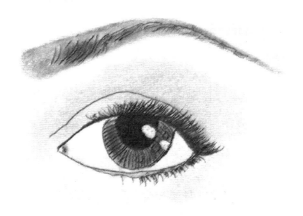

Step Four: Paint in faux hairs

Whenever there is a large area of missing brow I use faux hairs. If you have colored in the nasal edge (because the brows have been tweezed out) use faux hairs. If the arch is so thin you have had to paint on more than a sixteenth of an inch, you need faux hairs. If the tail is too short you need faux hairs. I am not suggesting every day. But when you want absolutely-undetectable-drop-dead-gorgeous-brows, do this.

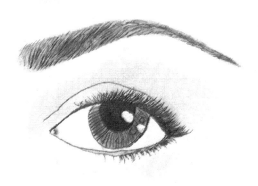

I wet a brow cake so it is saturated with water. I gently roll the tip of the brush against the surface of the cake. If the brush is pressed too hard, the tip will be muddy. I do it lightly so the tip stays pointed and wet. I stroke the brush against my palm so I can see what the load of the brush is. If the strokes look fine I proceed to the brow. If too thick, goopy or heavy, I rinse the tip and start over.

Before I put the eyeliner brush to the face, I observe the brow's natural growth pattern. That is what I recreate. If the natural growth is up and down, I follow it. If it slants right or left, I follow that. I also pay attention to the texture of the brow. Some darker, lighter, shorter, longer, thicker, thinner or whatever it takes to look real. This procedure does take practice but it works best.

When the steps are combined masterfully you will be amazed at how good you look. Sometimes I will use a little brow set or liquid brow tint to offset gray or wiry brows.

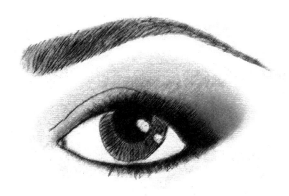

Perfect Brow with Eye Makeup

Beauty Communication

This is my fourth beauty book, my second,"**_I Want Your Face"_** in 1991 brought lots of attention to the art of eyebrow design. I think nearly every fashion magazine or makeup artist called me. I have had artists come from all over the world to study my techniques.

We all want to communicate as clearly as possible. To be successful in doing so, we need to understand that we communicate with our eyebrows as well. To the viewer brows that are droopy, thick, thin, too high or too low may give the wrong impression. Since brows are a key in beauty communication lets make them look as perfect as possible.

In beauty, communication is very important. But you can't say you communicated just because you spoke. You have to give the other person a context in which they feel comfortable to hear you.

I hear women say, "I told her just what I wanted, but look what I got."   If you are nervous or demanding or willful, the context for an artist to hear you is non-existent.

So it is very important that when you go to a beauty professional you are centered and in a calm place. If you are going somewhere to have a service and it's loud, overstated and distracting, I would suggest looking elsewhere. The same is true if you walk into a salon and instantly feel inferior, the place is not for you - at that time.

 At first, it may seem there are no places to go. But the right place will occur as you have a deeper sense of your real needs. When you have a deeper sense of yourself you are more comfortable within and with your beauty. It's a special self-communication. This oddly enough translates to a type of serene beauty.

A feeling of beauty will remain elusive as long as you allow yourself to feel flawed. It is not easy to overcome these feelings, but it can be done. Working on your look and perfecting it helps. The real transformation is gradual and must take place from within.

Beauty is knowing you look beautiful because you are. You were made beautiful. Nothing on this Earth that happens to you can change that, if you choose for it to be that way.

Being beautiful means letting go of control and letting things be. You must also let yourself just be. When you can be comfortable just being, beauty occurs. And wherever there is beauty, miracles happen.

Imagine if Cinderella had said to her Fairy Godmother, "Go to Saks, they have just the dress I want, it's Chanel. I really want to make my wicked step-mother feel like trash, she is so mean! Don't forget the shoes; they have to be Crystal not glass! And call Rolls Royce and get me the best car they have."

This paradigm is not the one we have come to know and love. Demandingness never comes from feelings of confidence or graciousness. It comes from insecurity, it certainly is not beautiful.

Knowing you are beautiful, allows you to show up with confidence. Confidence brings grace. Confidence elicits the spirit and your beautiful spirit is *The Hidden Heart of Beauty.*

Your Power to Change

How we react to information affects our power to influence it. Too often, women are overly sensitive to comments about their appearance. They become whiny and angry and that limits their capacity to create change.

Recently I was at a photo shoot. The model was beautiful, but her eyebrows had been whittled down to harsh lines. I corrected them for the photo and politely suggested she let them grow out. We shared a caring moment and she left.

As she was leaving I heard her telling her friend about my suggestion. The friend's reply was, "I don't let anyone tell me what to do. Just who does he think he is?" That answer is simple. I am the one who can make you beautiful.

It takes courage for me to tell a woman her look is not working. But I feel this way. I tell a woman the truth. I tell her in a safe space for her to hear it. I let her know I understand the thought process that brought about her vision of herself. I affirm her beauty even if I disagree with her perceptions.

I do not criticize, attack or blame. Some words hurt, other words heal. I am very careful of what I say and how I say it. Because if you are in a place where you are honored, you can feel gratitude. Gratitude is the essence of happiness. When you are happy you shine. When you shine you are confident. And when you get to that place you are in the most profound state of beauty. **You will be seen. You will be beautiful.**

In the years I have done my beauty miracles, I promise you, more than any other single thing; women have said over and over, "Your eyebrows really do it for me." "I can not believe the difference." "No one has ever done them better, ever." "I love the look and now I finally really get it!"

I acknowledge my gifts in this area and give thanks that so many women have taken the time to tell me so. I am also grateful that I have had the opportunity to make their lives richer, fuller, more beautiful and more confident.

Being Visible and Loved

I always want to be noticed. To be overlooked has always been the worst of all possible inevitabilities.

I have spent my life studying appearances, beauty, and the visual in its many forms. **How to be seen. How to be beautiful.** I have developed and perfected it with my own maturing. Shocking people is of no interest to me. I realize that what I want—what everyone wants—is to be loved. And to be loved is to be seen.

I have seen in myself what I see in others: how we cleverly distance ourselves from love with grooming choices. Most often, I see clients with hair and makeup that are not only not alluring, but that also discourage personal contact. What is disguised as glamour is really just a canny way of avoiding love. When we do a hard, sometimes chic presentation, it can take on the look of a female impersonator, not a person who wants intimacy with others.

Many women tell me they feel invisible.

What makes people visible? Confidence. Confidence is knowing what to leave in as well as what to leave out. Confidence is poise. Confidence is choices made with certainty, not whim. Confidence is a state of grace that is not demanding or willful.

But there is more to being visible: are you a person who absorbs the light or projects the light? People who are visible shine like beacons. They don't just tolerate others, they accept them.

People who project light attract others to them. You cast a spell by taking the time to shine: makeup, eyebrows, hair, nails, clothing, shoes, perfume, you do it all *well*. No matter where you go or whom you see your beam is at 100% and you look flawless.

If you are one who absorbs light, you often feel invisible. If you are busy spreading light you don't have time to feel invisible. Some people ask, "How do I shine light I don't have?" Well, everyone has that special light inside. Sometimes life choices dim it, but it never goes out. When a woman is young and beautiful and innocent she walks into a room and all the eyes are on her like a million flashlights.

She has no reason to do anything but absorb. But as time goes on, she walks into a room as a thirty, forty, fifty or sixty-something and unless she has perfected the art of beauty communication and looking her very best, the room can seem quite dark. At that point she would feel invisible.

I remember one woman who complained of feeling invisible. She wasn't going to wear makeup or put any real energy into a party she had been invited to. Well, trust me you never know who's watching you. So for a few minutes you put out some energy and show up looking great. This gives you practice for the real opportunities. There is no sense waiting for a door to open and not looking your best when it does.

Put out some energy and you are a magnet.

Many women I see at parties, socially, or around town have not changed their makeup. However they have tried to update their look with cosmetic surgery and a new wardrobe. You can have all the surgical procedures and wear chic designer clothes, but if your makeup is dated, you're dated.

I see it all the time. A woman will get lip augmentation, face lift, eye lift, a face peel, dermabrasion, or laser peel, and then apply the very same makeup.

A woman who goes to my gym spends a fortune on hair coloring and styling. She has spent even more to have her lips filled to look full and young again. She works out everyday, but I doubt she has ever bought a new lipstick or makeup base color.

Many women think nothing of spending $200 or more on a dress, but without the face to go with it they may as well leave the dress in their closet. Recently, this fact was made crystal clear at a glamorous costume party. I took my favorite girl friend, whose face I had made up in an exceptional glittery cat makeup. She wore tight fitting black trousers, a black turtleneck, and black ballet slippers. When we arrived at the gala, all the women had spent a king's ransom on elaborate costumes and wigs. But the paparazzi ignored them and repeatedly photographed the cat face that I designed. She was the most visible woman at the party with nothing more than a gorgeous face and a wonderful sense of fun!

This is all quite philosophical, but it's what has brought me to where I am today. I take makeup, clothing, hair and every aspect of grooming quite seriously. An actress friend once said, "You don't have to be on stage to be a star." I could not agree more. The world is a stage and you are starring in your own life. Show up and put out some energy! Know you look good because you have practiced. Show up 100%, that gives you confidence. **You will be seen. You will be beautiful.**

When you feel invisible is when you make poor choices and learn bad habits. You are simply reacting, and when in this mode you can't see clearly. So you look to experts. Well, I can assure you, you will never find one in the cosmetics department of any store. The people working there can't serve your needs because their goal is to sell their line of products. At BeautyBoyz our goal is to create beauty and that is what we do perfectly. So, come in and meet me personally. Let me give you what you never knew you could have.

Terminology

There are some terms one might want to know to make understanding Eyebrow Architecture easier. To avoid explaining positioning or crucial land marks over and over, understand the terms listed below.

- **Base Cutting:** This refers to cutting the brow hairs at the skin's surface. Micro scissors are laid flat to the skin and the hairs are cut invisibly at a level parallel with the skin. This enables one to remove unwanted hair and test a new arch pattern before any tweezing is done. This type of cutting also allows soft removal of tiny hairs around the brow that interfere with a clean looking brow line, arch, or highlighting.

- **Brow Cake:** This refers to a Cake Eyeliner that is water soluble. Cake Eyeliner is available in a variety of shades.

- **Canthus:** This is the junction where the eye opens and closes. There is one at each end of each eye.

- **Iris:** The colored part of the eyeball. The pupil is the black dot in the center of the iris.

- **Lateral:** This refers to the section or edge of the eye closest to your hairline. So the lateral edge of your eye would be the section that is from the outside edge of your iris to the lateral canthus.

- **Medial:** This refers to the section in the middle of the eye. For our discussions about eyebrows the medial area refers to the section that holds the iris of the eye. The iris is the entire medial area of the eye.

- **Nasal:** This refers to the section or edge of the eye closest to your nose. So the nasal edge of your eye would be the section on the inside edge of your iris to the nasal canthus.

- **Orbit:** The circular bone around the eye. This bone protects the eye. The top of this bone is what many refer to as the brow bone. The interior is referred to as the eye cage or eye socket.

- **Palpable Fold:** The fold of the eye. The crease of the eye. Most Asians are missing a palpable fold which results in a flatter appearance to the eye area.

- **Trimming:** This refers to trimming off long brow hairs. This can be done in three ways. Comb the brow hairs up and cut them off following the top contour of the brow. Comb the brow hairs down and cut them shorter following the bottom contour of the brow. Lay a brow comb parallel to the growth and cut off the excess length.

- **Tweeze:** Often referred to as the French Method. This means using tweezers to remove unwanted hairs to obtain your desired pattern.

- **Ventilate:** This refers to removing only some of the hairs in a dense brow to make it look softer. Example: This could be done by tweezing out every other hair or trimming out every other hair.

- **Waxing:** This refers to a method of applying wax to the area where hair removal is desired. A muslin (or special paper) strip is pressed into the wax then pulled off for a very clean finish. This method is good for wide areas but not next to the exact arch line. Wax tends to spread and remove hairs under the growth line that make the brow look artificial. This is primarily due to the position of the patron when the wax is applied. It is also common to "eyeball it" and make a mistake. The mistake would be ending up with eyebrows that don't match.

Fun Brow Stuff to do yours perfectly every time

- *White Pencil*

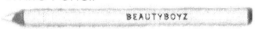

- *Tweezerman Tweezers*

- *BBz Micro Scissors*

- *Medicon Surgical Scissors*

- *Eyebrow Groomer Brush/Comb*

- *30/0 Fine Eyeliner Brush*

- *Brown or Black Cake Brow*

- *Blonde or Taupe Brow Pencil*

- *Brow Shaper Trio:* wax center, with two brow shades on either side.

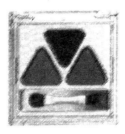

- *Slant Brush,* stiff bristle: used with both wax and powder.

- *Alabaster Primer:* used to highlight the lower contour of the brow.

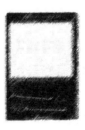

- *#12 Neutralizer Brush*: used to apply Alabaster Primer.

David's Bio

In the realm of cosmetic artistry, David Starr is *the* superstar. David began his solo makeup career in 1973 in LA. He opened his first San Francisco studio in 1984—it was the first ever self-contained makeup studio. It was so successful that in 1989 a group of clients bought him a billboard overlooking Union Square and put up his photo with the caption reading, Unequalled Makeup Artist.

His catchphrase "I Want Your Face" was on everyone's lips. Then he developed his own line of cosmetics with then shockingly innovative names like Hussie Black, Wicked Wife, Die My Darling and Seduce & Abandon. Then in 1991 he wrote the best selling book *I Want Your Face*. His salon continued to flourish and became one of those legendary places the press loves. David was named best makeup artist in SF by Harper's Bazaar in 1987 & 1988. Best Makeup Artist by San Francisco Magazine and The Nob Hill Gazette in 1988 & 1989. He also received the Doer's Award for being one of the most influential people in San Francisco. He has been seen in every top fashion magazine, including, London's Tattler, Vogue, Allure, Mademoiselle, Cosmo, Bazaar, Elle, In Style...and on and on. In 1994 a New York financier made him an offer he couldn't refuse to buy out his lease.

He sold it and he moved to Palm Springs, where he continued developing products, writing, touring and lecturing in New York, Dallas & San Francisco.

In 1999 he partnered with financial wizard Ed Russell to form an LLC called BeautyBoyz. They have kept the best of David Starr Beauty and developed a new line of Mineral Makeup called BeautyBoyz.

David does not focus on superficial appearances. His clients adore him because he is a "Makeup Psychologist "and he helps them strengthen their confidence & self-esteem. Today a global community of women can take advantage of David Starr & the BeautyBoyz through their website, lecture tours and in-house makeup lessons. David is best described by a favorite client, "He's a hellava nice guy with a wicked sense of humor."

David Starr and the BeautyBoyz have been seen in;

Vogue, Allure, Mademoiselle, Cosmo, Bazaar, Elle, W, In Style, Tattler, Palm Springs Life, Hwy 111, Muscle & Fitness, Good Housekeeping, First for Women, San Francisco Focus, SF, San Francisco Magazine, Nob Hill Gazette, San Francisco Examiner, San Francisco Chronicle, The Desert Sun, Desert Woman, Desert Post Weekly, and others....

Dedication

Some friends who have inspired me, stuck with me, listened to me, and loved me as I have loved them.

Connie Francis, **Barbara Towery**, Miss Joey English,
Stewart Weiner, *Erik Sandoval*, Joyce Jaber,
Dee Danna, Janice Battaglia, Heidi Ellsworth, Loraine Palmer,
Betty Barker, Pam Price, Linda Boyce, Lisa Baxter Cobler,
Beverly Clevenger, Connie Russell, Pattie Daly Caruso,
Marilyn Delfs, Janet Newcomb, Pam Hinnant, Anilise Hyllmon,
Florence Goldby, Mary Louise Kirch, Janet Kleinberg,
Gina Luciano, Debi Valentino, Shirley Van Bibber, Jorie Parr,
Diane Marlin-Dirkx, Geneva Tice, Tina Wong,
Amy Antinetti, Megan Hahn, Patti Gribow, Linda Austin,
Harley, Cindy Santoscoy, Heather Davis, Sharron Stroud,
Joyce Dougherty, *Eric Akin*, Tiffany Duck, Hon. Cheryl Mills,
Peri Wolfman, *Dr. Sheila Newton*,
and
**The First Lady of the Entire Coachella Valley,
Miss Jackie Lee Houston.**